ABOUT VITAMINS

In this age of processed foods it is becoming increasingly more important to ensure that our diets provide us with an adequate supply of vitamins for the maintenance of good health. This book, an introduction to the subject, serves to dispel any misconceptions that may exist and recounts the fascinating story of man's discovery of nature's keys to radiant health.

ABOUT VITAMINS

Nature's Keys to Radiant Health

by

P. E. NORRIS

THORSONS PUBLISHERS LIMITED
Wellingborough, Northamptonshire

First published 1960
Second Impression 1962
Third Impression 1964
Fourth Impression 1967
Second, revised Edition 1969
Second Impression 1970
Third Impression 1972
Third Edition, revised and reset, 1975
Second Impression 1977
Third Impression 1979
Fourth Impression 1980

ISBN 0 7225 0307 5

Filmset by
Specialised Offset Services Ltd., Liverpool
Made and Printed in Great Britain by
Hunt Barnard Printing Ltd., Aylesbury, Bucks.

CONTENTS

CHAPTER ONE

ABOUT VITAMINS

The oddest ideas exist about vitamins. Most people imagine that all one has to do is to take enough of the right kinds of vitamins to render one immune to coughs, colds and all the other ills to which man is heir. This idea was encouraged by a spate of misleading advertisements.

It is as well, therefore, to know something about vitamins; what they can achieve and what they can't; in which foods they exist, and whether natural or scientifically conjured vitamins are best.

One dictionary defines vitamins as substances, the chemical nature of which are imperfectly known, present in food in their natural state, of man and animals, derived originally from plants, and essential to health and life, deficiency or lack of which causes diseases such as beri-beri, rickets, scurvy, etc.

The odd thing is that no one knew anything about vitamins about 65 years ago; the very name did not exist. Then, why, you may be tempted to ask, if man existed tolerably well for 10,000 years without vitamin supplements, is it necessary to be worried about them now?

There are at least three reasons:

1. In one part of the world or another men have always been afflicted by scourges like beri-beri, pellagra, scurvy and rickets, even in the midst of plenty, without being able to account for or cure such diseases, and only relatively recently have scientists realized that there was some missing factor from foods which caused them;

2. With the increase in population and the decrease of arable land and the animal manure that kept it fertile, a good deal of food is now processed, with a resultant deficiency in vitamins and essential minerals. Vitamins can, however, be produced in the laboratory but there is a world of difference between natural vitamins (food concentrates) and synthetic vitamins. The Russians carried out tests which proved that synthetic vitamin C is less effective than vitamin C from natural sources, or in the form of food concentrates, and this doubtless holds good for other vitamins as well.

3. With the rapid advance of scientific knowledge, the discovery of vitamins, their sources and uses, vitamin therapy was almost automatic.

For centuries physicians, sea captains and explorers have suspected that when food lacked certain substances scurvy would attack men. For decades they searched blindly for cures. Captains Cook and Lind were pioneers.

In 1882 Admiral Takaki of the Japanese Navy, thought he had found a cure for beri-beri; as long ago as 1865, A. Trosseau laid down in the *Standard Treatise on Medicine* that cod-liver oil was a perfect cure for rickets; in 1838 another Frenchman, Jules Guerin, propounded the theory that rickets was a deficiency disease; and in 1889 Bland Sutton used cod-liver oil to relieve lions in the London Zoo of rickets. De Gouvea, physician on a Brazilian plantation, was puzzled by workers who could see well in daylight, but not in the dark.

But neither these nor any other investigators knew exactly what there was in lemons, for instance, that cured scurvy; in the foods that relieved beri-beri; in the cod-liver oil that rid lions of rickets; or in the green leaves that caused those who were night-blind to see. Men were groping and guessing.

How changed is the scene today. All but the veriest tyro knows about vitamins and can rattle off their names and acquaint you with the diseases they cure.

Early Discoveries

When discoveries started to be made they occurred simultaneously in different countries as a number of men got on the track of these missing factors, which, if added to food, cured dread diseases. Such men as Eijkman, Lancaster, Kramer, Holst, Frolich, Funk and Hopkins.

At first it was thought that there was but one elusive element which, if added to food, would act as a panacea for all deficiency diseases. One who almost hit the bull's-eye was Lunin, a pupil of Professor Bunge, at Basle, who after hundreds of experiments on laboratory animals came to the conclusion that they would not survive if fed indefinitely on a diet of purified fat, protein, carbohydrate, salts and water; that is, all the known food constituents.

He said: 'A natural food such as milk must therefore contain besides these known principal ingredients, small quantities of other and unknown substances essential to life.' His results were tested and confirmed by scientists both in Europe and America.

Dr Stepp, a German, got even closer to the solution. He fed mice on bread and milk from which he removed the unknown element essential to life. Many of his mice collapsed and died, but he was able to cure some who were in dire straits, by putting back that 'alcohol-or-ether-soluble substance indispensable to life.' But no one knew precisely how to isolate the substance.

Hopkins went a step further. He fed mice on

proteins, carbohydrates, fat, milk and yeast and found that half a teaspoon of milk added to a synthetic diet made all the difference between life and death to his animals. If milk were not given, yeast had the same effect.

The story of vitamins, their discovery and isolation reads like an exciting detective story. One clue after another came to light – some purely by chance – till the solution was laid bare. Then how simple it seemed.

In 1912, Casimir Funk, a Pole, and Sir Frederick Gowland Hopkins, simultaneously published statements on 'anti-beri-beri vitamines' and 'purified diets' respectively, which aroused immense interest in scientific circles. Their labours were complementary.

Hopkins impressed physiologists with the exact, quantitive nature of his experiments; Funk was the first actually to isolate a vitamin, though he stated in error that beri-beri, scurvy, rickets and pellagra were all due to 'vitamine' deficiency.

Years earlier Eijkman had shown that beri-beri could be controlled by 'something' contained in the thin red husks that surround grains of rice before polishing, and in 1911 Funk succeeded in extracting from rice polishings a crystalline substance which in fact cured beri-beri. This is now known as nicotinic acid.

The Word 'Vitamine'

When analysed these crystals revealed the presence of nitrogen in basic combination; that is, the so-called 'amine' nitrogen. And with true scientific logic Funk decided that as the substance was a life-giving one its name should start with the prefix 'vita', meaning 'life'; and on to this he tacked the suffix 'amine', and so the word 'vitamine' was born.

In 1913, when Dr E.V. McCollum was working with Dr M. Davis at Johns Hopkins University, they also discovered a growth-factor in butter and egg yolk. This was not an 'amine', so yet another name had to be found and it was called 'unidentified dietary factor, fat-soluble A', or, as we know it now, vitamin A.

Scientists had shown that yeast also contained the same 'vitamine' that exists in the rice husks, so Funk set about trying to isolate a similar crystalline substance from yeast. He obtained 200 lb of yeast and continued to reduce it in search of the elusive crystal, till eventually he ended with one-twelfth of an ounce of the crystal.

It wasn't very long before scientists and doctors realized that all deficiency diseases could not be cured by the same 'food accessory'; that pellagra did not react to the vitamin that cured scurvy and that victims of scurvy felt no relief if treated with the vitamin that cured rickets.

Slowly, brick after brick was added to the wall, but even now the structure is by no means complete, though it presents a formidable barrier to most deficiency diseases.

There are still dreadful ailments that resist every drug, food and vitamin, or other treatment: rheumatism, arthritis, arterio-sclerosis, disseminated-sclerosis, polio, haemophilia, etc. In some, pain can be alleviated and a minor degree of improvement obtained, and it is possible that eventually such diseases will respond magically to undiscovered hormones or vitamins and that broken and racked bodies will recover as they did in the past in cases of pellagra, beri-beri, rickets and scurvy. Who knows? All we can do is work, delve and hope.

Organic Chemical Compounds

Vitamins are not elements in a chemical sense, for an element 'is a substance which cannot by chemical processes be broken up or separated into substances of different nature from itself.'

They are organic chemical compounds and when Funk invented the name 'vitamines' he did so in the belief that all vitamines were nitrogenous compounds allied to the 'amines'. When it was proved that this was not so, the final 'e' was dropped.

Later, when Szent-Gyorgi first prepared the anti-scorbutic vitamin which now bears the title C, he believed it to be a sugar, and since the names of all sugars end in 'ose', suggested that it should be called 'ignose'.

After the first ten vitamins had been isolated it was known that they were compounds with little in common as far as chemical structure is concerned. Some are sugar acids; some sterols; some contain nitrogen; some no nitrogen at all. They are not foods because they do not keep hunger at bay and exist only in minute quantities.

Because not all the vitamins were discovered simultaneously (even now new ones are being unearthed) the units by which they are measured are different. The original unit of vitamin C, for instance, was the least amount of the vitamin that would prevent the development of scurvy in a pig! And the first unit of vitamin D was the amount needed to secure what was called two-plus healing in the bones of a rickets-stricken rat. Later D was expressed in Steenbock Units, Poulsson Units, A.D.M.A. Units and rat units.

Then the League of Nations established a Nutrition Section, which appointed a committee to decide on a uniform standard, and today, vitamin measurements have been standardized. A and D are expressed in i.u.'s (international units) and the remainder either in milligrams or micrograms.

Not a Cure-all

Before I go any further let me warn readers that vitamins are not 'cure-alls'. They are *not* a substitute for good wholesome food, and they will *not* guarantee you against colds, coughs, pneumonia, measles, influenza, baldness and housemaid's knee. They protect only if you eat the right food and live the proper way. You can't break all the rules of sound living and keep fit just by taking vitamins.

Remember, also, that some vitamins deteriorate if exposed to air, heat or light; that storage for long periods renders others valueless, especially if not kept in sealed, airproof containers.

In my opinion it is preferable, by far, to eat foods in their unrefined state and so get the minerals and the vitamins that accompany them, and benefit thereby.

Recent legislation has made it obligatory for manufacturers of vitamins to state on the labels of bottles the exact strength of their products, though they need not say whether the vitamins are natural or synthetic – a significant omission.

Having warned you and said all the unpleasant things I can think of about vitamins, let us now see what they *can* do for you.

CHAPTER TWO

VITAMIN C

Men in olden times should not have suffered from
deficiency diseases for vitamins abound in an endless
variety of foods, and, if absent in one, they were
almost certainly to be found in another. Moreover,
they lived out in the fresh air and light so their bodies
should not have lacked vitamin D.

But on long ocean voyages and in countries in the
far North, where green stuff is scarce in winter, they
suffered from the oldest of deficiency diseases – *scurvy*.
It is so unpleasant a disease that it gave its name to a
deceitful type of behaviour and we speak of those
who act in an underhand way as 'scurvy knaves'.

Most people have not seen and will never see a
case of scurvy, for though our civilized mode of living
has added many diseases to the already long list,
there are some that have been conquered, and scurvy
is one of the worst.

If a diet lacks fresh fruit and vegetables, scurvy will
develop after 4-6 months. It was once thought to be a
skin disease and people shied away from scurvy
victims as if they were lepers, for it affects the skin,
the walls of the blood vessels, gums, teeth and bones,
and makes its presence felt gradually and insidiously.

First there is a feeling of intense fatigue, which is
not relieved by sleep; then headaches and a chronic
disinclination for work. Nature paints dark rings
under the eyes; joints and limbs start to ache and
swell – which symptoms are sometimes mistaken for
rheumatism – tiny haemorrhage spots appear round
the hair follicles on the legs or where there is friction

from clothing. If limbs are pressed, they bruise. Later, the muscles bleed, the nose bleeds and limbs pain when moved because of the weakness of the walls of the blood vessels. Gums become soft and spongy and resemble fungoid growths; they ulcerate and bleed; the breath grows foetid and eventually teeth loosen so that they can be plucked out by the fingers. Bones become brittle and fracture easily; finally – unless there is a drastic alteration in diet – death overcomes the victim.

No wonder that hardened mariners who drank, fought and took life without shrinking, quailed at the thought of scurvy.

Men who sailed on long voyages realized that they were risking death, for if they did not reach their destination in four or five months they would fall to the scourge and would soon be too weak and helpless to work their ships.

Limes and Lemons

Many cures were tried and rejected before seafarers realized that in lemons they possessed a certain cure. Even then they did not know why. It was not until 22 April 1927, that King George V signed a document which states that 'Whereas by Section 200 and the Fifth Schedule of the Merchant Shipping Act, 1894, power is given to His Majesty by Order in Council to make provision as to the use of anti-scorbutics other than lime or lemon juice of such quality and composed of such materials and packed and kept in such a manner and served out at such times and in such quantities as His Majesty may direct ... '

According to His Majesty's direction, concentrated orange juice can now be used provided 'it shall not contain less than 70 per cent of total soluble solids by weight, shall be free from signs of alcoholic fermentation and contain no mould growth. It shall be so prepared and stored that there is no material loss of vitamin potency.'

Centuries ago men knew that there was some essential principle in fresh food that enabled them to resist scurvy, so, before they embarked on long voyages, loaded as much fruit and vegetables as possible. But vessels were tiny, cargo space limited and they did not know which foods were best.

It is said that Hippocrates was the first to describe scurvy, but that is doubtful. It is a disease that does not touch the Mediterranean countries where fresh food abounds and where seamen are rarely more than a week's sailing distance from a coast. The first genuine descriptions date from the thirteenth century, and later Anson, in his account of his voyage round the world, describes how his men were attacked by it. Admiral Richard Hawkins says that within his experience 10,000 seamen died from scurvy.

More than one galleon was found adrift, every man dead – all victims of scurvy! When Vasco da Gama rounded the Cape of Good Hope in 1498 he lost no fewer than 100 of his crew of 160.

When Jacques Cartier visited Newfoundland for the second time in 1535 his crew suffered so severely from scurvy that 100 out of 103 were incapacitated and 25 died. When the ship touched land they crawled ashore and erected an image of Christ, before they prostrated themselves, chanting litanies and singing psalms. But this availed them not at all.

Cartier then observed that a native who had been down with scurvy was about and well, so questioned him and learnt that the leaves of a certain tree were an effective remedy. It proved to be sassafras. A decoction made of the bark and leaves was given to his men and the effect was miraculous. James Lind wrote, 'it wrought so well that if all the physicians of Montpelier and Louvaine had been there with all the drugs of Alexandria, they would not have done so much in one yere, as that tree did in six days.' Though the experience was recorded, the lesson was not assimilated.

More than three centuries later, during the Alaska gold rush, an American, Dr Sidebotham, found himself with a number of scurvy-ridden patients, but with no antidote. Nor is there any green vegetation in Alaska in winter, except pine needles. So he pounded these, made a mixture with water and administered it to his patients, who recovered rapidly. Later it was proved by laboratory tests that pine needles contain as much vitamin C as orange juice. It is unlikely that they will be used elsewhere, except, perhaps, in Russia, where they are experimenting with them.

Early Mistakes

A cure for scurvy was not discovered earlier because men were led astray by false reasoning. In the Low Countries, where scurvy seems to have been prevalent in the sixteenth century, one of the foremost Dutch physicians, Forestus, had his own antidote. After administering it he used to send patients inland to a healthier atmosphere, for he put the condition down to fogs, damp soil and sea mists. They journeyed inland, ate fruits and fresh vegetables and, naturally, were cured. But both the patients and the learned doctor imagined that a change of air had worked the miracle.

Doctors thought that 'sea scurvy' and 'land scurvy' were different diseases, though the symptoms were identical.

All sorts of theories were put forward to account

for the disease. John Gerard, author of the famous
Herball, said that the disease attacked 'such as
delight to sit about without labour and exercise of
their bodies.' Hawkins was sure that 'change of aire
and untemperate climates' were the causes.
According to him it was caused by prolonged
exposure to sea air; and he, being an experienced
mariner, was heeded.

His men never suffered from scurvy, it is true,
when they ate plentifully of 'sowre Oranges and
Lemons', but then they were usually ashore when
they ate fruit; thus he was convinced that of all
remedies 'the principall of all is the Ayre of the Land;
for the Sea is Naturall for Fishes and the Land for
Men.'

In 1600 the cure was nearly found. On 13
February four ships left Woolwich for the West
Indies and crossed the tropic of Capricorn on the 24
July after putting in at the Canaries. Many were
stricken by scurvy on three of the ships, but on the
Commander's ship the crew were in sound health
because he had taken aboard bottles of 'the Juice of
Limons, which hee gave to each one, as long as it
would last, three spoonfuls every morning fasting;
not suffering them to eate any thing after it till noone.
The Juice worketh much the better, if the partie
keepe a short Dyet, and wholly refraine from salt
meate, which salt meate and long being at Sea is the
only cause of breeding this Disease.'

On the strength of this the East India Company
ordered all its captains to maintain a supply of lemon
juice on their ships. The Dutch East India Company
went further; they ordered their captains to load
fresh fruit and established a vegetable garden at the
Cape for the benefit of ailing seamen.

Then a mistake was made that put the clock back.

These early voyagers were convinced that it was the *acidity* of the lemon juice that kept scurvy at bay, and they reasoned that *all acid fruits and vegetables were good*. So they are. But they made the terrible error of substituting acid food of every kind for lemons. They didn't realize that it was the vitamin C that cured; they thought it was the *acid*.

So some doctors recommended vinegar; others diluted vitriol! (sulphuric acid). Why men continued to pin their faith in such deadly poison for more than a century is difficult to understand. Even Sir Richard Hawkins considered it a sound remedy, if less effective than lemons. 'The Oyle of Vitry,' he writes, 'is beneficiall for this disease: taking two drops of it.'

Now that we know how simple it is to cure scurvy one looks back with amazement at the hit-or-miss methods to master the scourge. No one tackled the disease scientifically.

In Britain few, except the very poor and those in prisons, had scurvy, so there is some excuse for the belief that it was caused by the excessive use of salt meat.

Herbal Remedies

In ancient times herbalists abounded and their remedies included oranges, lemons and oil of vitriol for seamen; scurvy grass, brooklime, cresses, parsley, chervill, lettuce, purslane, winter rocket, strawberries and a multitude of herbs and berries.

The Diary of John Manningham (1602-3) gives Dr Parry's popular remedy: 'Of the Juyce of Scouruy-grasse one pint; of the juyce of water-cresses as much; of the juyce of succory, half a pint; of the juyce of fumitory, half a pint; proportion to one gallon ale; they must all be tunned up togither.' Perhaps the ale had something to do with its popularity.

Gradually it dawned on men that lemons and oranges were the finest medicines and that fresh vegetables helped. In 1878 Dr T. Trotter wrote in *Medicine Nautica: an essay on the Diseases of Seamen*, that scurvy broke out among slaves on the Guinea Coast, who were fed on boiled beans, rice, Indian corn and palm oil. When they reached Antigua the master was able to buy limes and lemons and soon every one of the 300 slaves aboard was restored to health.

In all it is estimated that no fewer than ten million slaves perished, mainly from scurvy, while being transported from Africa to America and the West Indies.

In 1753 James Lind wrote *A Treatise of the Scurvy*, the most comprehensive study of the disease ever made, and four years later the Lords of the Admiralty issued a rule that all ships were to be victualled with lemons and fresh vegetables.

Captain James Cook used sweetwort, sauerkraut and lemons, though he and many others lost faith in lemon juice because, when stored, the vitamin C is likely to vanish. They did not, of course, know this, but only that it failed to cure victims of scurvy.

Sir Gilbert Blaine was another who believed that fresh meat, vegetables and fruit were effective in curing scurvy and it was on his recommendation and that of Dr Blair that the Admiralty finally adopted lemon juice as the main anti-scorbutic and ordered that one ounce of juice with an ounce and a half of sugar was to be issued daily to each man after six weeks at sea. The results opened men's eyes. In 1760 there were 1,754 cases of scurvy in the Naval Hospital at Haslar; in 1806 there was only one!

Though scurvy was conquered, the principle which relieved men of the disease was neither known nor understood. Nor do all living creatures react in the same way to the same foods. Captain Cook observed, for instance, that whereas sheep, goats, pigs, monkeys and guinea pigs suffered from scurvy; rats, cats, birds and dogs did not.

This is because rats and birds have the faculty of making vitamin C from some substance in their food; and we have since learnt that cows also manufacture their own vitamin C.

Scott of the Antarctic

Though it could be cured, men did not realize that vitamin C was the magical essential missing from foods in order to resist scurvy, and in 1912 when Scott set out for the South Pole he firmly believed that fresh meat was a good anti-scorbutic, so loaded up with plenty of meat and what he thought were good strengthening foods.

Of one supper he wrote in his diary: 'We had four courses; the first pemmican (without vegetables), full whack, with slices of horse meat flavoured with onion and curry powder and thickened with biscuit; then an arrowroot, cocoa and biscuit hoosh sweetened; then a plum pudding; then cocoa with raisins, and, finally, a dessert of caramel ginger.'

Onion and curry powder contain some vitamin C, but this was destroyed by cooking. The other edibles had none.

Scott's team ate plentifully of thick soups, meat, fish, porridge, bread, butter, cake, biscuits, jam, fruits, jellies, seal steaks and mutton. 'We are living extraordinarily well at base,' wrote Scott. 'Under the circumstances it would be difficult to conceive more appetizing repasts or a regime which is less likely to produce scorbutic symptoms. I cannot think we shall get scurvy' (!).

His medical advisers were to blame. Didn't they

know that lemon juice would have saved every man? Hadn't they studied the history of scurvy?

Amundsen was better advised. At his base 350 miles away he prepared differently for his 850 miles trip. 'It was our aim,' he said, 'all through to employ fruit and vegetables to the greatest extent; there is undoubtedly no better means of avoiding sickness. Previously the pemmican had contained nothing but the desired mixture of meat and lard; ours, besides, had these vegetables and oatmeal.'

Courage and physical stamina are of no avail, as Scott's unfortunate men discovered, if not fed properly. When Scott's men succumbed there was only a distance of 11 miles between them and safety. Had his rations contained sufficient vitamin C history might have been written differently.

The 'Kronprinz Wilhelm'

The finest of so-called strengthening foods will endow the body neither with strength nor vigour unless microscopic quantities of vitamin C are present. The case of the ocean raider 'Kronprinz Wilhelm' is a classic example of this and should be better known.

On 11 April 1915, she made for Newport Mews on the Atlantic coast of America, where her crew was interned; not because she was defeated in battle but because 110 of her complement of 500 were prostrated by what the doctors thought was beri-beri, but which was really scurvy. Newspaper men were barred from the vessel.

Learned discussions took place between medical men ashore and the ship's doctors, but they could agree about neither the cause nor the cure. Then came an interruption. A launch drew alongside, a man bearing a card showing that he was a famous scientist climbed aboard and was admitted to the discussions. Suddenly one of the doctors cried, 'Why — that man is McCann of the *New York Globe*!'

Before they could hustle him off the ship McCann admitted, 'Yes, I have used a card that does not belong to me; but I was also Chief of the Bureau of Chemistry under Dr Harvey W. Wiley and I know a good deal about dietetics. Hear what I have to say.'

He hadn't spoken for five minutes before the ship's surgeon, Dr E. Perrenon, rose and extended his hand. 'I welcome you, Mr McCann, and I will hear what you have to say when these gentlemen leave.'

McCann learnt that the ship had been at sea for 255 days; that there was an abundance of food, most of it taken from liners the raider had sunk. From the 'Indian Prince' she had stocked her larder with meat, white flour, margarine, canned vegetables, cheese, coffee, soda and biscuits. A month later 'La Correntina', with 5.6 million lb of fresh beef aboard, was sighted. Before sinking her the Germans took all the meat they needed. In turn, 'Bellvue', 'Anne de Bretagne', 'Mont Angel', 'Hemisphere', 'Highland Brae', 'Wilfred M', 'Samentha', 'Guadelope', 'Tamar' and 'Coleby' disgorged their holds for her benefit.

For months the Germans lived like lords; then suddenly the crew started to complain of pained and swollen limbs, fatigue, disinclination to work and other symptoms of scurvy. They would not respond to medical treatment.

'Though 110 are in the sick bay,' said Perrenon, 'the remainder are on the verge of collapse. We could not work the ship, but had to make for port.'

Perrenon did not know of the work of Scandola, who had demonstrated that nothing promotes the elimination and loss of calcium more than decalcified foods such as white bread, white sugar, meat and refined corn; nor of the researches of Drennan, who proved that when calcium is withdrawn there is fatty infiltration and fatty degeneration of the liver. The blood refuses to coagulate, scratches bleed profusely and haemorrhages occur even in the long bones.

Medical men knew less about diet than they do today, but McCann had studied the effects of food on human beings for half a lifetime and knew that denatured food caused most illnesses. He told Perrenon about his work, and the German agreed to carry out his instructions.

'Leach 100 lb of bran in 200 lb of water,' ordered McCann, 'for 12 hours at 120° F. Drain off the liquor and give each man 8 oz. every morning, as well as a tablespoon of bran morning and night.

'Boil cabbages, carrots, parsnips, spinach, onions, turnips together for two hours. Drain the liquor and discard the residue. Feed this soup in generous portions with unbuttered wholemeal bread.

'Wash and peel potatoes. Throw away the potatoes, but boil the skins and give each man 4 oz. of the liquor daily.

'Every day each man must have the yolks of four eggs beaten in raw unskimmed milk – one egg every three hours. In addition, give them orange and lemon juice; apples and apple sauce. No man must touch denatured food such as he has eaten in the past $8\frac{1}{2}$ months.'

By 16 April ten more had fallen ill; thereafter there were no new cases, and on 19 April four were well enough to go on deck and others showed signs of improvement. On the 21st eight were dismissed from hospital; on the 22nd eight; on the 23rd four; and on the 24th seven. One man who had been completely paralysed could stand! In ten days 47 were passed as fit to work and eventually every man was restored to health.

No drugs were given, but all fat, egg albumen, cheese, meat, white flour and white sugar were withdrawn from their diet.

Were the results of this cure noised far and wide? NO. Perrenon was ordered by Count Bernstorff, the German Ambassador, to suppress all facts concerning conditions aboard. Did the American Government, then, give the case national publicity? Again, NO.

Full details were submitted to Surgeon-General Blue and he, Dr Arthur H. Glennan, Acting Surgeon-General, and Dr J.W. Kerr, Chief of the Research Laboratory, did their utmost to broadcast the story, but failed. The milling, sugar-refining and other interests who spend millions of dollars annually de-naturing foods, were too powerful. The story would never have become known but for McCann.

What is Vitamin C?

This and other examples have been given to show what happens when there is a lack of vitamin C. But you will also want to know how it acts; what it does, and in what foods it exists.

Vitamin C produces and maintains intercellular material which cements individual cells into a tissue or organ functioning as a whole. Without enough vitamin C the entire bodily structure is affected; the blood vessels become porous and let the blood through; muscles weaken. and may even grow paralysed; mineral salts drain away from bones and teeth; cartilages grow so weak that they won't hold the joints together; the walls of the lungs cave in; anaemia develops in the cells of the bone marrow, tissues degenerate and wounds refuse to heal.

The dentine or bony material between the root canals and outside enamel of teeth is produced by cells called odontoblasts. If the body lacks vitamin C these shorten and become separated from the dentine by fluid; the dentine becomes porous and in the case of children the teeth refuse to grow; they develop fissures and cracks which house decay. Gums become spongy, but if treated with 50 mg of vitamin C the condition will be cleared up within two weeks.

Unfortunately, vitamin C is the most unstable of all vitamins and is destroyed by heat, light and exposure to air, and most of our common foods: meat, bread, milk and all dried or preserved foods, contain little or no vitamin C. In the past canning methods destroyed every iota of the vitamin, but today canners of tomatoes and fruit juices have developed techniques which preserve most of it, so that canned orange, lemon, tomato and other juices are fairly good sources.

Sunlight on ordinary glass bottles robs milk of 79 per cent of vitamin C, whereas, if placed in brown glass, the loss is only 1.3 per cent. On the advice of scientists the Danish government decided that all milk in Denmark will be sold in brown glass bottles. Stiff wax-paper cartons in which milk is sometimes sold in Britain, serve the same purpose.

The potato contains some vitamin C, which exists not in the skin, but in the interior, so that much is retained in the cooking – especially if baked in its jacket. The skin retains the mineral salts, the interior the vitamin, and as most people eat a good deal of potato they get a fair share of the vitamin. In the last century the potato was Ireland's staple food and when potato disease devastated the crop in 1845-46, deficiency diseases struck down thousands, who died from scurvy and a dropsical condition known as hunger-oedema.

If only they had known that all the vitamin C needed to cure them was 1/500th of an ounce daily!

No international agreement has been reached as to the vitamin C requirements of the human body, and there is still some confusion as to the quantity needed daily. The British standard is about 30 milligrams, whereas in the United States it is twice this, and much larger quantities have been recommended by various experts. Dr N.N. Yakolev, member of the Academy of Sciences in the U.S.S.R. reckons that the vitamin C requirements of Olympic athletes is about 400 milligrams a day. Some authorities say that one milligram per pound of body-weight is safest.

C is the vitamin we should worry about most because not only is it unstable, but it cannot be stored in the body and drains away rapidly under conditions of cold, heat, fatigue and stress, this last a condition from which millions more suffer today than at any time in the past.

Best Sources
Rose-hip juice is the richest of all known foods in vitamin C, with an average of 520 mg of the vitamin in 100 g ($3\frac{1}{2}$ oz.) of the juice; black currants 231 mg, parsley 176 mg, paprika 160 mg, kale 145 mg, horseradish 136 mg, Brussels sprouts 112 mg, turnip tops 100 mg, asparagus tips 98 mg, cabbage 90 mg, strawberries 61 mg, orange juice 58 mg, lemon juice 46 mg, red currants 46 mg, grapefruit and pineapple juice 40 mg, tomatoes 24 mg; but every fresh green vegetable and fresh fruit contains some C. Of flesh, only raw liver contains an appreciable amount and even fresh meat is remarkably poor in vitamin C.

When food is cooked much of this vitamin is

destroyed. Pressure cooking affects it, too, and the addition of soda or the use of copper utensils kills every vestige.

No one need ever go short of vitamin C, even in winter, for grass contains 350 mg per lb weight, far more than orange juice, and watercress is another excellent source. But dried fruits, legumes, dried peas and similar foods don't contain any.

Milk, an excellent food in other respects, is a poor source, rendered poorer by pasteurization, and if again subjected to heat all vitamin C vanishes.

If you think that you're not getting enough, drink the diluted juice of one lemon every day or 3 oz. of orange juice. When canned there is no significant loss of C in fruit juice – even if chilled – but if fruit is cut with a steel knife or stored for lengthy periods there is a gradual loss of vitamin C. When making salads, break lettuces and other green leaves with the fingers instead of cutting them.

Don't imagine that any old diet plus a little synthetic vitamin C is an adequate substitute for a good, well-balanced diet of milk, eggs, cheese, fresh fruits and vegetables and wholemeal bread. It isn't.

Though no one need go short of vitamin C, thousands do, unfortunately, mainly through ignorance or poverty. Old Age Pensioners who exist mainly on white bread, margarine, jam, tea and other foods lacking in vitamins A, B-complex and C, often suffer from mild scurvy which does not incapacitate, but enervates and opens the door for other illnesses.

CHAPTER THREE

VITAMIN A

Some vitamins, like C, are soluble in water; others like A, in fat. This is one of the first things scientists discovered about them.

Lack of any vitamin impairs the efficiency of the body, but lack of vitamin A rarely results in a disease that incapacitates the victim or prevents him from earning a living.

The scientific name for this vitamin is axerophthol, and it exists in plants in a yellow pigment called carotene, which is converted in the animal body into a nearly colourless compound.

So far two kinds of vitamin A have been identified: one in the livers of salt water fish, called A1; the other in the livers of fresh water fish, called A2. Scientists have proved also that an enzyme or ferment in human liver converts the provitamin A (carotene) into active A1 or A2. There is also some evidence that a similar conversion may take place in other organs or tissues of the body.

You may read advertisements which claim that vitamin A is an 'anti-infective vitamin', and will immunize the body against colds, which makes some buy the vitamin and ignore the normal rules of health. Such advertisements should be taken with a large pinch of salt.

A, like all the other vitamins, tends to make bodily tissue resistant to germs, but only if you maintain a healthy regimen. In children, lack of vitamin A results in retarded growth and imperfectly formed bones and teeth, and though adequate doses of vitamin A will not guarantee immunity from colds and similar infections, it will help to make children healthier and more robust.

The function of vitamin A is to keep healthy the epithelium or linings of mucous membrane throughout the body. If these are not maintained surfaces grow rough and horny – keratinization is the technical term for the condition – and fail to secrete sufficent fluid.

The conjunctiva of the eye becomes affected as well as the linings of the respiratory, digestive and urogenital tracts. They become clogged with lifeless, horny cells in which all sorts of dangerous micro-organisms flourish.

In birds the feathers are affected; in animals the fur; and both human beings, as well as animals, suffer from a peculiar and characteristic eye disease.

Night Blindness

One result of a deficiency of vitamin A is night blindness. Some time ago a man driving fast on one of our arterial roads was stopped by a police car, and the officers asked him what he meant by driving on the wrong side of the road and accused him of being drunk. He was escorted to the station, but there was no evidence that he had taken even the smallest quantity of liquor. He confessed, however, that he found it difficult to pass cars coming towards him, and admitted that he drove mainly by instinct! 'The lights dazzle me,' he confessed.

When sent for a medical check they found that his skin was dry and flaky, his hair brittle and falling, and an oculist discovered that he was completely blind in the dark! He confessed that each time he entered a darkened cinema his wife had to guide him to his seat. But none of these facts was known to the licensing authorities simply because they didn't ask for them. So this menace was allowed on the roads at night, when keen sight is more than usually needed!

Doctors discovered also that he ate practically no fresh vegetables, dairy products or fish, but existed mainly on meat, potatoes and bread. Large doses of vitamin A were prescribed and he was told to eat generously of greens. In *a few days* his night-sight improved astonishingly.

The authorities in the United States say that 10 per cent of their drivers suffer from night blindness, and the rate of recovery from momentary glare-blindness is now the basis of tests for vitamin A deficiency.

Night blindness has been known to the medical profession for centuries and the Chinese, Egyptians, Greeks and Romans all cured it by eating liver. Hippocrates advised his patients to eat the liver of an ox (raw), with honey, daily.

It is possible, however, to imbibe too much vitamin A. Eskimoes in Greenland refuse to touch the liver of the polar bear, which contains such enormous quantities that it poisons both men and beasts; even huskies will not eat it.

Red Indians eat the adrenal glands of the moose, which are rich both in vitamins A and C; and Laplanders the contents of the reindeer's stomach, together with tiny shoots, moss and leaves it may contain, for the same reason.

Xerophthalmia and Keratomalacia
In areas of the world where poverty is rife and diet lacks variety people suffer from eye diseases due to lack of vitamin A, and to other diseases due to a dearth of the B-complex vitamins. In 1939 the Committee on Nutrition in the Colonial Empire published a report

which stated: 'Diseases caused by deficiency of vitamin A are perhaps the most common in all the Colonial Empire. There are reports from a wide selection of territories of affections of the eye, night-blindness, xerophthalmia, keratomalacia ... '

During the First World War when the Germans commandeered all the butter and most of the green vegetables they could lay hands on in Denmark, Dr Hinehede, who was in charge of nutrition, placed the nation on a diet of potatoes, root vegetables, rough rye bread and skim milk. They thrived and the death-rate fell lower than it had ever been; but because the foods lacked vitamin A (present in butter and greens) many went blind.

The remedy, of course, was plenty of fresh raw milk, butter, cod-liver oil and green vegetables. Ten grams of cod-liver oil daily will cure xerophthalmia, or dry eye, in just over a week, but the antidote came too late for thousands of Danes.

In children the symptoms of this disease are stunting of growth, apathy and wasting; and in all, diarrhoea, bronchitis, pneumonia, catarrh and discharges of pus from nose and ears, and in the urine. Very unpleasant indeed.

Much the same thing happened in Rumania in 1918. People were forced to live mainly on maize meal and soup concocted from bran and root vegetables, and thousands turned blind. The Austrians had stolen their cattle and the cod-liver oil which might have saved them was brought into the country much too late by Dr Gideon Wells.

Where there is a shortage of rich milk, cod or halibut-liver oil, or green vegetables, we find xerophthalmia. It is rife among the poor in Brazil, in parts of China, the Dutch East Indies and the lush island of Ceylon, and McCarrison saw thousands of cases among impoverished Indians.

Much despised grass is a rich food and may one day supply us with most of the nutriment we need. Grass contains 28 times more of all the vitamins, except D, than all other vegetables, and powdered grass is a highly concentrated protein food. In 1918 when the Austrian Army occupied the Northern Italian village of Auronzo they took away so much food that for a whole year the 5,000 inhabitants were forced to exist mainly on hay and the luxuriant grass in the mountains. During that period there was not one death in the village and all kept exceedingly fit, but when after the war they returned to normal food, the death rate was frightful. During that year there were no cases of xerophthalmia.

This disease has afflicted man for centuries. In 1842 Dr Budd, lecturing on 'Diseases Arising from Defective Nutriment', cited cases of ulcerated cornea which occurred among people on restricted diets, and explained how they could be cured by animal food. Dr W. Mackenzie also noted how rife xerophthalmia was among the poor in 1847.

In the same year Dr David Livingstone recorded that members of his expedition in Africa suffered badly with their eyes when they lived for long periods exclusively on manioc meal and coffee. 'Eyes become affected,' he wrote in his diary, 'as in the case of animals fed in experiments on pure gluten or starch.' As a medical missionary, Livingstone was trained to notice such signs and act on them.

Shortly after the Second World War tests carried out in the United States showed that 50 per cent of normal children and adults were mildly deficient in vitamin A, and of those admitted to hospital five per cent had a serious deficiency.

Many adults suffer from a vitamin A deficiency, but

because the symptoms are not painful or crippling, they are unaware of it. Often no notice is taken until they start to grow blind. Blindness from such cause is unnecessary and can be prevented by doses of 2,500 i.u.'s of vitamin A daily. This is the equivalent of two milligrams of carotene or 1/50,000th of an ounce, and can be provided by one pint of milk, an egg, one ounce of butter or a large helping of greens daily.

Most newly-born babes have a low vitamin A reserve and as mother's milk is not rich enough to build this up quickly, vitamin A concentrates are sometimes prescribed. Nursing mothers should also be sure that their diet contains sufficient of this vitamin.

How the Eye Reacts
As few know anything about either the chemistry or mechanism of sight and there is very little written for the layman on the subject, it may be of interest to explain how it is that you see.

The eye sees when the light rays are focused on the retina of the eyeball by the lens, just as in a camera. The retina corresponds to the sensitive chemical layer on the plate or film of a camera.

A snapshot by a camera cannot be seen until the film is developed, and similarly the eye cannot see till the impression on the retina is developed. The picture on the retina is developed by nerve impulses which travel from the retina over the optic nerve to the brain, and something there translates them into vision. The full process has still to be explained.

In a photographic film the image is formed by chemical changes in the film; usually by a change of silver salt to silver. Much the same thing happens in the eye, where the pigments involved are stored in the rods and cones of the retina. In the rods there is stored a pigment called *visual purple*; in the cones,. *visual violet*.

When rays of light strike the visual purple they bleach it to a yellow substance known as *retinene*, which produces nerve stimulus. Once visual purple has been bleached it will not respond again to the stimulus of light until it has been changed back into visual purple and this cannot be accomplished unless there is an adequate store of vitamin A in the body. There are other reasons why visual purple cannot be restored, but lack of vitamin A is the most common. and important. Visual violet is similarly affected.

The first to connect sight affliction with a lack of green foods was De Gouvea in 1883 when he was doctor on a plantation in Brazil. He noted that though the slaves could see perfectly all day, they could not find their way home in the dark. After much investigation he decided that their diet lacked sufficient green food, and when green leaves were added to their meals, their night-sight was restored. This was long before any of the vitamins were discovered.

Almost all diseases are caused either by a lack of essential foods or a faulty balance of diet, for food nourishes the blood, and blood, propelled to every part of the system, enables limbs, muscles and organs to function efficiently. If the blood has a tendency towards acidity, or if its flow is restricted in any part, trouble follows. It is on this foundation that the science of Osteopathy rests, by which so many ills that have baffled the medical profession have been cured.

Sources of Vitamin A

Now a few words about some of the foods that contain vitamin A. It is found in all green vegetables;

those with green or yellow leaves are richer than those with white. The outer green leaves, usually discarded, are richer in carotenoids than the blanched ones inside; green celery and asparagus contain more than the bleached varieties. Yellow potatoes contain some vitamin A; white ones do not.

Parsley is a rich source and an ounce in weight of fresh parsley will supply your needs for one day, but as many vegetables and herbs contain the vitamin, there is no need to stuff on parsley. Dandelion leaves also provide this vitamin, and can be eaten in salads or cooked.

Many of our richest greens, such as nettles, can be found in fields and hedges but because they are free, people spurn them. If your doctor prescribes vitamin A, you can save extra expense at the greengrocer or chemist by rooting out dandelion from your garden.

Halibut-liver oil is the richest known source, for $3\frac{1}{2}$ ounces contain 100,000 i.u.'s, and one drop about 3,200 i.u.'s. One teaspoon of cod-liver oil contains 3,500 i.u.'s, $3\frac{1}{2}$ oz. of egg yolks 2,800 i.u.'s; but if you eat generous helpings of greens (cooked) or salads every day, you will obtain enough. In fact, almost every food has some of the vitamin.

Exposure to heat and air tends to destroy vitamin A and carotene, but if there is heat only and no air, the vitamin is unaffected. Consequently, though $3\frac{1}{2}$ oz. of milk contain only 110 i.u.'s, the values for evaporated and dried milk, which are far more concentrated, are 670 and 875 i.u.'s respectively.

Because there is so much vitamin A in so many foods the risk of deficiency is small if the diet is a varied one. If you imbibe more vitamin A than you require for immediate needs the excess is stored in the liver, so if a reserve is built up you can live for some time without an additional intake. However, excessive dosages of this vitamin serve no useful purpose, and in extreme cases can be dangerous to health.

CHAPTER FOUR

VITAMIN D

Vitamin D should be of special interest to the British, who see so little sun. It is erroneously called the 'sunshine vitamin', as most people imagine that the sun's rays contain vitamin D. This is excusable as rickets, for instance, is cured by the aid of sunshine as well as by taking vitamin D in some form.

Rickets was once the scourge of the English. In 1645 Daniel Whistler, a student at Merton College, Oxford, wrote a thesis on the subject. In 1650 the famous Dr Francis Glisson, then a professor at Cambridge, gave for the first time a detailed description of the symptoms of the disease which throughout Europe was known as the 'English Disease'.

Rickets must have been rife not only in Britain but all over Europe. C.C. and F.M. Furnas say in their work *Man, Bread and Destiny* that the infant Jesus in the better-known paintings of the Madonna and Child, has legs bearing all the symptoms of rickets! Yet the artist must have accepted his model as a normal child of the period.

The first to connect sunlight with the cure of rickets was Dr T.A. Palm in 1890. He pointed out that as far as he knew, wherever there was plenty of sun, rickets was absent and his researches showed that the skeletons of Egyptian mummies were free from it.

About that time a Dane named Niels Finsen sat by
an open window watching a cat on a roof below. As a
shadow of a wall moved slowly over the cat it rose
and moved into the sun. Each time the shadow
overtook it, the cat moved further out. 'Why,' asked
Finsen, 'does a cat so crave the sun? Isn't the fur,
which keeps it warm in winter, protection enough?'

Finsen, who was born in Iceland and trained for
medicine in Denmark, came of a race where men are
taught to think for themselves. Cats, he reasoned, are
rarely ill. Sunlight therefore, is not an element that
merely keeps them warm. It contains something that
keeps them fit.

So he read all that he could about sunlight, and
learnt that the ancient Egyptians, Assyrians, Chinese
and Greeks healed some ailments by sunlight; that
the Incas and natives of India cured skin disorders by
exposure to the sun; but that in Europe in the Middle
Ages exposure of the body — and bathing — were
considered ungodly.

He learnt that a French doctor had cured ulcers
by exposing them to sunlight, and wounds and
tumours by reflecting the sun's rays on to them
through a lens. In 1815 Loebel of Jena constructed a
box made of glass into which the sick were placed,
called heliothermos, which wrought wonderful cures.

Finsen experimented on himself by painting a two-
inch band of Indian ink on a forearm and exposing it
to the sun. In three hours the entire arm, except the
inked portion, was red and sore.

He reasoned that there was something in the black
pigment that prevented the sun burning his arm,
though it did not prevent it from growing very warm.
From this he deduced that there is a pigment in the
skin of dark and sun-browned people which protects
them from sunburn. Later, when his arm grew

brown by constant exposure he found that it did not
burn and peel if exposed for long periods. From this
he concluded that skin absorbs something from the
sun's rays and stores it in the body; some protective
pigment.

In 1893 he conducted experiments both with pure
sunlight as well as sunlight through lenses. He found
that the sun had beneficial as well as harmful effects;
that if patients with smallpox were exposed to
sunlight the blisters festered and their faces remained
scarred; but if they were shielded by red curtains
that let in the red rays and kept out the chemical
blue, violet and ultra-violet, no scars remained.

Finsen made hundreds of experiments and
founded the sciences of heliotherapy and
phototherapy; he cured by quartz light, X- (and
other) rays, and his work was carried on by others,
most notable of all, Dr Rollier of Leysin, whose
sanatorium became world famous.

Doctors knew that exposure to sunlight cured
rickets. They did not know why, and this puzzled
them. One of the facts they did learn, however, was
that the dark-skinned are more prone to rickets than
those with fair skins.

Cod Liver Oil

In the nineteenth century cod-liver oil, that nasty
elixir, was considered a remedy for a number of
ailments. In his *Journal* Arnold Bennett wrote that an
omnibus driver told him: 'I've driven these roads for
eight-and-twenty year, and the only pal I've found is
cod-liver oil. From September to March I takes it
and I never has colds nor nothing o' the sort. I give it
to my children ever since they were born and now
I'm blest if they don't cry for it.'

Fifty years ago mothers gave their children castor

oil and cod-liver oil at the slightest provocation.

Everything having failed, the English surgeon, Bland Sutton, tried cod-liver oil on monkeys, lions, birds and bears suffering from rickets in the London Zoo — and they recovered! Apparently there was something that sunlight ·and cod-liver oil had in common. But what?

In 1906 Gowland Hopkins spoke of rickets as a disease of which 'we have for long years knowledge of a dietetic factor', the real error being 'to this day quite obscure'.

In 1915 Edward Mellanby at Cambridge found that cod-liver oil and other animal fats (known to contain fat soluble A) protected puppies against rickets, so that for some little time it was thought that the 'unknown factor' was contained in vitamin A.

It was not till 1919, however, when rickets became more prevalent in Berlin because of the scarcity of food, that a German-Jewish physician, Huldchinsky, tried to cure the disease, not by natural sunlight, which was often absent, but by ultra-violet rays. Cures were rapid and permanent as long as the ray therapy continued. In 1924 two Americans, Hess and Steenbock, irradiated food with ultra-violet rays and, with it, cured rats suffering from rickets.

Ergosterol

By now it was known that rickets could be cured by (1) sunlight; (2) cod-liver oil; (3) ultra-violet rays; (4) food irradiated by ultra-violet rays. Finally it was proved that it was in *sterols*, waxy materials associated with fats in food, that the vitamin was present. But, in which *sterol*?

As the best known is cholesterol, it was thought that the anti-rickets vitamin was the same as irradiated cholesterol; but tests showed that this was not so and that the true pro-vitamin must be some *impurity* present in cholesterol.

Many experiments and tests were made before it was decided that ergosterol (ergot-sterol, because it is derived from ergot, a fungus that grows on rye) was the parent substance of vitamin D.

The next step was to isolate the pure vitamin from ergosterol. This was more difficult than scientists imagined for when ergosterol is irradiated, many similar substances are formed alongside one another, all so much alike that they can hardly be distinguished from each other.

Eventually, in 1932, pure crystalline vitamin D was isolated simultaneously by Dr R.B. Bourdillon and his colleagues in London and Professor Windaus and his colleagues in Gottingen, and all medical men agree that in the cure and prevention of rickets synthetic vitamin D is more useful and convenient than cod-liver oil.

The vitamin D in fish oils is identical with the vitamin D in ergosterol when irradiated by ultra-violet rays.

Ergosterol is known as vitamin D_2; vitamin D in cod-liver oil is known as vitamin D_3, but as D_2 and D_3 are equally effective they are marked on bottled vitamins merely as D so as not to confuse the public.

Pure vitamin D, which is also found in many foods in their natural state, in infinitesimally minute quantities, is 400,000 times more potent than cod-liver oil and according to Dr L.J. Harris, a tablespoonful of cod-liver oil (a suitable daily dose for a child) contains less than a millionth of an ounce of the pure vitamin. One ounce of pure vitamin D is therefore enough for a million children!

D is one vitamin of which you can have too much for 500-1,500 i.u.'s will prevent rickets, 1,000-3,000 i.u.'s will cure it; and 10,000 i.u.'s is a toxic dose.

When the body has too little vitamin D, calcium and phosphorus are not absorbed through the walls of the intestines into the blood (from which they are passed on to build bones and teeth) but are excreted out of the body. So, *unless growing children are given enough vitamin D*, much of the calcium in milk and greens is lost, and bones become soft and bend, and teeth break down. Once the adolescent stage is passed, the lack of vitamin D is less serious.

Healthy Teeth

Because milk is rich in calcium, milk plus adequate amounts of vitamin D are more effective than milk alone.

In the twenties two Americans, Boyd and Drain, noticed that every one of 28 children admitted to hospital for diabetes, suffered from dental caries, but after a period on a strict diabetic diet, all caries were arrested. They then tried this diet on children with decaying teeth who were not diabetics and again all decay was arrested in ten weeks. The significant items in that diet were one quart of milk, one egg, two large helpings of vegetables, six teaspoons of butter and one teaspoon of cod-liver oil daily.

They improved on this diet by substituting vitamin D milk for ordinary milk, and twice the amount of cod-liver oil.

As long ago as 1918 Mrs (later Lady) Mellanby realized that vitamin D helped to prevent children's teeth from decaying, and on her evidence P.G. Anderson, C.H.M. Williams, H. Halderson and C. Summerfieldt, carried out an experiment on children in two orphanages in Toronto in 1932. Both groups were given a. diet generous in milk, meat, eggs, vegetables and fruit and for one year they were made to live out of doors whenever the weather allowed. They were also made to brush their teeth daily.

At the end of the period it was found that each child had an average of 1.5 new cavities in his teeth, whereas children in other schools in Toronto had three cavities.

Each orphanage was then divided into two groups; one received eight drops of viosterol (1,000 i.u.'s of vitamin D) every day in a ginger cookie; the other a cookie without the vitamin. It was found that between the ages of 3-10 the vitamin had a marked effect in preventing decay; after that the effect was diminished.

From these and similar experiments we have learnt that vitamin D given in the formative years builds strong teeth, sound bones and lays a foundation that cannot be put down after puberty.

Daily Needs

Vitamin D is still necessary after that age, but a sufficiency can easily be obtained from milk, butter, eggs, fresh green vegetables, fish oils and, of course, is made in our own bodies and with the aid of sunshine and LIGHT.

Nursing mothers and growing children need more vitamin D than adults. Infants two-three weeks old should have 350 i.u.'s a day; during the second month 700 i.u.'s; until puberty 1,000 i.u.'s as well as a quart of milk.

Adults need 200 i.u.'s daily as well as a pint of milk. There is vitamin D in milk, but this varies tremendously with pasture and the manger in which the cow lives. The sunnier the country, the richer the milk *should be* in vitamin D, though if the cow is lodged in a cellar or tied in some dark, narrow passage-way, as is sometimes the case in the East, its milk will be almost devoid of vitamin D.

The Importance of Light

According to Dr Vaughan, *light* is an important factor — not merely sunlight.

Incidentally, ultra-violet rays will not penetrate ordinary window glass or a garment made even of the flimsiest material. The skin itself must be exposed. Special glass, which it is claimed will allow the ultra-violet rays to pass, is only 66 per cent effective.

Dr Vaughan found not a single case of osteomalacia among the rude, rough boatwomen who live in houseboats in the Kashmir Valley and exposed vast areas of their bodies. They also ate plentifully of fresh vegetables, drank raw milk and worked hard.

According to Dr Rollier of Leysin, the skin is the *most important organ of the body*, for it controls and stimulates every metabolic process and, if deprived of light, cannot function normally. This is why the Ancient Greeks were so fit, even girls exercised naked in the open.

From all this you might conclude that sunlight contains vitamin D and that by mysterious means conveys it into our bodies. That is not so.

Almost every fresh food we eat contains some trace of this vitamin which is stored in the body, but not used. It exists in the skin in a provitamin condition. When the sun's rays strike the bare skin the *ultra-violet rays* activate this provitamin and vitamin D passes into the body cells. Even now we don't know exactly how this happens.

One can imbibe too much vitamin D. If you take too large a dose of sunshine the skin is burnt and you may even become poisoned. Too much sun on the back or the back of the neck can result in sunstroke. If excessive doses of cod-liver oil, halibut-liver oil,

ergosterol or other forms of vitamin D are taken,
some form of bone calcification may result.

We know a great deal about vitamin D and the
good it can do; but not all. Like vitamins A and C it
stimulates and aids the healing of wounds; it has
been used successfully to treat some cases of asthma
and hay fever, whereas other cases of the same
complaints are made worse by it! Why?

Vitamin D has been used for treating a distention
of the cornea of the eye, known as keratoconus; but
there is so much that we don't know and research is
continuing so fast with this as with other vitamins,
that discoveries changing the whole nature of vitamin
therapy may take place within the next ten years.

CHAPTER FIVE

THE B-COMPLEX

The B family is the most confusing of all the
vitamins. What was thought to be one vitamin, now
turns out to be many. B_1 is known as thiamin in
America and aneurin in Britain; B_2 or G is known as
riboflavin; P-P is nicotinic acid, known as niacin in
America; B_6 is pyridoxine; then there is B_3, B_4, B_5,
Filtrate Factor or Pantothenic Acid; B_7 or vitamin I;
H or Biotin; J; Anti-Grey Hair Factor; B_{12}; Factors
L_1 and L_2; Factor M; Factor W; and Grass Juice
Factor.

In this work we shall deal mainly with B_1, B_2 and
nicotinic acid, and touch on B_{12}.

Vitamin B_1
As both B_1 and C are partly destroyed in the body
and passed out in the urine, supplies must constantly
be replenished. The body will not store B_1 as it does

A or D, so if living far from centres where foods containing B1 can be obtained, it is as well to stock with synthetic B1 vitamins.

If there is a serious shortage of B1 there will be (1) loss of appetite or craving for unnatural foods (birds and animals eat their feathers or their own excreta); (2) indigestion, diarrhoea alternating with constipation and possibly colitis (inflammation of the colon or large bowel); (3) lassitude and loss of weight; (4) headaches, a tendency to dropsy, and rough, unhealthy skin; (5) sub-normal temperature, palpitations and heart trouble.

These early symptoms grow much worse if the body continues to be deprived of the vitamin, and when there is an absolute dearth of vitamin B1 the state known as beri-beri is present. Legs grow numb and calf muscles painful, the entire body becomes emaciated and partly paralysed, and there is a peculiar kind of heart trouble in which the right side of the heart grows enlarged and the rate of beat rises.

Sometimes, instead of becoming emaciated, the body swells with water. This is known as 'wet beri-beri, and unless B1 is given in large doses, the patient will die.

Beri-beri is mainly a disease which afflicts poor, rice-eating peoples who have little with which to supplement their rice; and it is probably a disease of recent origin — since the polishing of rice became universal.

At first Orientals with traditional fatalism accepted this as an Act of God, but the Director-General of the Japanese Navy, K. Takaki, did not. He rightly decided that beri-beri was caused by a lack of some substance in the diet, so when in 1882 the training ship 'Ruijo' set out on a nine-months' cruise and 169 cases of beri-beri developed among his crew of 276, of whom 25 died, he pondered long over the disaster. When, soon after, a second training vessel, 'Tsukuba', was sent on the same course, Takaki saw to it that the diet of her crew was changed.

He believed that beri-beri was caused by a lack of protein so reduced the quantity of rice and added meat and milk to the rations. During the cruise, which lasted ten months, there were only 14 cases of beri-beri and the only members who developed the disease were those who had refused the new diet.

This was a triumph for Takaki, who further increased the amounts of meat, fish, milk, and fresh vegetables in the diet and cut down the rice. Takaki was made a baron for his services.

A Dutch doctor in Java, named Eijkman, was not, however, satisfied with Takaki's solution. In 1897 all the fowls he used for experiment were struck down by a disease identical with beri-beri, but which in fowls is called polyneuritis.

'How did the fowls get this disease?' Eijkman asked. On enquiry he learnt that they had been fed on polished rice left over from the hospital kitchen. He then fed them on unhusked rice and they recovered with incredible rapidity.

Each grain of rice is surrounded by a husk, which, being unpalatable and inedible, is removed. The grain itself wears a thin coat, either white, red or yellow – occasionally black; very much like the thin skin on a peanut. It is this skin that is removed by polishing between rollers covered in sheepskin so that 'table' rice emerges white and 'refined'. It is this skin which also contains the valuable vitamin B_1.

Eijkman was vitally interested. He continued to poke and pry, visited 27 prisons and found that beri-beri was rampant wherever polished rice was eaten, and in some prisons as many as 50 per cent of the inmates were down with the disease. In every instance wherever rice wearing the thin skin was fed to the prisoners they recovered speedily.

This did not prove Takaki wrong in giving added meat, fish, vegetables and milk to his sailors, for vitamin B1 is also present in much smaller quantities in those foods, for neither Takaki nor Eijkman knew anything about vitamins.

In 1908-9 two English doctors, Frazer and Stanton, fed coolies suffering from beri-beri on unpolished rice and cured them. Major Chamberlain of the U.S. Medical Corps, stationed in the Philippines, read about the results achieved by the Englishmen. Of the 5,000 men in his charge 618 had beri-beri, so in 1910 he substituted unpolished rice and beans for the polished rice in their rations, and the result was miraculous. In 1911 he had three cases; in 1912 two; and in 1913 none!

It was then discovered that yeast, which also contained this hitherto unidentified food factor, yielded even more startling results, so Funk set out to isolate the vitamin in yeast, and, as related, started with 200 lb and ultimately tracked down the elusive vitamin in crystalline form. All he got from 200 lb of yeast was one twelfth of an ounce. Since then it has been found that only 1/15,000th of an ounce of vitamin B1 is sufficient to cure paralysed pigeons of beri-beri within a few hours.

In 1912 an experiment was carried out in Billibid Prison, Philippine Islands, where 26 men were under sentence of death. Drs R.P. Strong and R.C. Crowell got the authorities to agree to substitute long terms of imprisonment for the death sentences if prisoners would consent to take part in food experiments.

They were fed exclusively on refined and

denatured foods, mainly polished rice. After six weeks there were signs of anaemia; water-logging and swelling of feet and ankles, which vanished when they lay down; weak and painful legs; puffiness under the eyes; swelling of the thighs and muscular weakness. Finally, the prisoners' hearts grew feeble — all signs of what was then known as 'prison oedema'.

These 'guinea-pigs' were allowed to mingle freely with the other inmates, but the condition was not contagious. When ultimately they were on the verge of collapse they were given natural brown rice, which quickly restored them to health.

The Nerve Vitamin

Is there some connection between vitamin B1 (and perhaps other vitamins) and paralysis of every kind? For B1 has been called the 'nerve vitamin', and lack of it tends to cause paralysis.

Without a doubt there is, though we don't know precisely what. In 1910, when infantile paralysis, or, as it is now commonly known, poliomyelitis, was almost unknown, a severe epidemic struck the Island of Nauru in the Pacific. In a fortnight 700 of the 1,500 on the island were laid low and 38 died.

Half those struck down were Nauruans, but natives from the neighbouring Carolines also suffered. Europeans on the island, however, were almost immune and the Chinese completely so.

Examination of the food of the Nauruans and Carolines showed that it was seriously deficient in vitamins, chiefly B1. Europeans ate food more plentiful in vitamins, and the Chinese diet was rich in green, fresh vegetables, for they are excellent market gardeners and their crops are cultivated in compost made up of wastes and night-soil.

Once the Nauruans used to quaff immense

quantities of yeast-laden beer, which provided them
with vitamin B1, but the sale of this was banned by
law.

Ultimately the authorities were forced to forbid the
sale of white flour and polished rice to the Nauruans,
at which there was an almost magical improvement
in their condition. Infant mortality fell from 50 per
cent to 7 per cent; leprosy and tuberculosis, which
were rife, disappeared, and there were no further
outbreaks of poliomyelitis!

Dr W.J. McCormick of Toronto, learnt of the
tragic events on Nauru and set about investigating
infantile paralysis in his home town. He questioned
50 polio victims and found that 33 ate no bread other
than white, and the other 17 ate white bread
regularly and brown — not necessarily wholemeal —
occasionally.

One polio patient attended by Dr McCormick was
a 14-year-old boy in Guelph, Ontario. He went down
with acute poliomyelitis, fever, headache, vomiting,
sore throat, stiff neck and pains in arms and legs on
15 October, 1938. Five days later he was taken into
Toronto for treatment and after five days of vitamin
B1 therapy, muscle pains, which were so severe that
codeine had to be administered, were eased and then
disappeared. On 7 November he was discharged,
being completely free from any signs of polio.

Dr McCormick's theory did not meet with general
acceptance by the medical profession, who pin their
faith in vaccines and injections. He believed that
polio and similar diseases are the final stages; that
such diseases make gradual inroads, unseen and
barely felt, for months and perhaps even years,
before the fatal stage. Lack of B1 is not the only one
which tends to cause paralysis; others, too, have
similar effects, namely B2, B6 and E.

White sugar, refined flour and polished rice should be banned by law. W. Addison, formerly Acting Provincial Commissioner, Central Province, Sierra Leone, wrote to the *Daily Telegraph*: 'Your columns report that vitamin B, prepared from rice polishings ... is employed in the treatment of beri-beri. But why encourage the production of polished rice?

'In Sierra Leone, many years ago, it was proved that rice as "cleaned" by the African women for human consumption, was nutritious and prevented beri-beri. It was also proved that human beings became inefficient when polished rice formed the chief food. As soon as "country" rice came into use efficiency was restored.

' "Country" rice formed part of my food for 20 years, as prepared and cooked by Africans. In "cleaning" rice in Sierra Leone, which, by the way, produces some of the finest rice in the world, much of the vitamin-containing covering was left on their grain, only the husk being entirely removed.

'Why go to the expense of removing health-giving parts, leading to further expense in preparing vitamin B for the cure of suffering which need not happen were nature not obstructed and hindered by "civilized, modern, progressive, refined methods"?'

I have harped a great deal on rice because it is in rice-eating areas that hundreds of millions suffer when rice is polished. The main sources of B1 are, however, natural wheat germ and yeast, and it exists as well in such products as yeast extract and in insignificant quantities in beef extract, which is not a yeast extract.

Because bran and 'middlings' are removed in the manufacture of white flour, wholemeal bread should always be eaten. It is the only bread with an appreciable amount of B1. Rye bread is also a good source, and, other fair sources are dried peas, lentils, nuts (not coconut), egg yolk and liver.

Nicotinic Acid

Next on our list is P-P (pellagra preventive), nicotinamide, or nicotinic acid, known in America as niacin. It is the recognized cure for pellagra, a disease you will never see if you live all your days in Western Europe.

Pellagra is a deficiency disease which in America attacks those who subsist exclusively on the three M's – meat, maize and molasses. We meet pellagrins in plenty in the pages of the works of men like Erskine Caldwell.

In 1915 no fewer than 11,000 Americans in the Deep South died from pellagra; in 1917, 170,000; in 1927, 120,000. Between 1915-16 it ranked second as the cause of death in Carolina and the Metropolitan Life Insurance Company stated that between 1911-16 more people perished in America from pellagra than either tuberculosis or malaria.

Why people in civilized countries should still succumb to pellagra is a mystery, for both cause and cure are known. The causes are the three M's; the symptoms the three Ds – dermatitis, diarrhoea and dementia. In the final stages it destroys the nervous system as ruthlessly as either beri-beri or polio.

The United States is not the only country where pellagra is rife; it is common wherever maize forms the staple food: Italy, Egypt, Rumania (before the war), South Africa.

The skin of the pellagrin becomes dark and bronzed like deep sunburn, symmetrically on each side of the face or body; on the backs of the hands or on the forearm. The skin roughens, cracks, becomes pigmented and loses elasticity, and it is from these symptoms that the affliction gets its name: 'pelle' (Italian for skin); 'agra' (rough).

The tongue swells and grows sore and the hydrochloric secretion of the stomach, which is needed for the digestion of proteins, diminishes. Thus, indigestion and constipation are among the early symptoms; with diarrhoea and the passing of mucus and blood later.

The nervous system is attacked and the pellagrin suffers from headaches, mental depression, insomnia and acute lassitude and melancholia. In the final stages he may toy with the idea of suicide.

It is one of those insidious diseases which develop so gradually and have symptoms which resemble so many other diseases that victims do not realize they are in the grips of pellagra till immobilized by cramp, wasting of muscular tissue, impaired vision and, finally, paralysis. At the end the pellagrin resembles a mummy whose bones try to push through taut, unhealthy, yellow-black skin.

Like scurvy and beri-beri, pellagra was once considered an infectious disease because the skin took on so repulsive an appearance. Those unacquainted with pellagra cannot be blamed if they edge away on seeing a victim for the first time.

A pioneer investigator into pellagra was Dr Joseph Goldberger, son of Hungarian emigrants, who went to New York in 1880, where they ran a grocery store in East Side. Goldberger became a doctor and at the turn of the century was paid to inspect immigrants on Ellis Island.

Later he was sent by the U.S. National Institute of Health to the South to investigate a new disease, pellagra, which was killing scores and incapacitating and sending thousands insane. When Goldberger reached the area he found that people were terrified of the disease, which they thought was contagious. He decided it was not.

It struck him as odd that none of the medical staff caught the disease, so deduced that pellagra may have been caused by faulty diet. On probing he found that the staff were eating a far more varied diet than the victims, who existed on corn bread, 'grits' and fatty pork.

He tried to give himself pellagra by scratching his arm and putting pus from pellagra sores on the scratches, but failed to get it. His colleagues thought that pellagra was due to lack of protein and few would listen to his theories.

Then Goldberger had a brainwave. He obtained permission for a squad in Rankin Prison Farm, a section of the Mississippi State Penitentiary, to be kept on a diet which he thought would bring about pellagra, and arranged for the volunteers to be pardoned at the end of the experiment.

The volunteers were fed on a diet of refined foods and at the end of five months six developed skin lesions typical of incipient pellagra. Others on the same food, but with the addition of a little milk, butter, lean meat and eggs, did not. When the pellagrins were given milk, butter, meat and eggs, they, too, recovered.

This convinced Goldberger that pellagra was a deficiency disease caused by eating refined foods, but he did not know exactly which substances were lacking and when he died in 1929 of a tumour of the kidney, the world was not much wiser.

In 1920 another American, the physiologist Voegtlin, cured pellagrins by giving them extracts rich in vitamin B (at that time thought to be a single substance), which cured them, but when he gave

them an extract made from the thin husks of rice (B_1)
it had no effect. This puzzled him.

In 1927 Goldberger had a similar experience, so
tried to find out whether there was some principle in
vitamin B which cured pellagra and another which
cured beri-beri.

For a few years scientists groped in the dark, then
between 1933-34 Kuhn, Gyorgy and Wagner-
Jauregg experimented with a substance called
lactoflavin, later renamed riboflavin (B_2), which they
hoped would cure pellagra, but found that though it
helped rats to grow, it did not do what they expected.

Eventually in 1937 R.J. Madden, a student of Dr
Elvehjem at Wisconsin University, remembered that
years ago Funk, who suggested that pellagra might
be caused by a vitamin deficiency, had extracted a
crystalline substance called nicotinic acid from
vitamin extracts, which he fed to polyneuritic
pigeons, but at the time little notice was taken of his
experiments. Madden tried nicotinic acid on dogs
with 'black tongue' (sore mouth), and it cured them!
So Madden, Elvehjem, Strong and Woolley wrote a
paper on their experiments; and almost
simultaneously Harriet Chick and Sir Charles
Martin in London, Fouts and Spies in the U.S.A.
and Hassan and Harris in Egypt tried it on humans
and all three groups were successful. The world was
then sure, for the first time, that pellagra had finally
and conclusively been conquered.

It is caused by a famine in the body, of nicotinic
acid. If the system is merely short of, but not
completely denuded of the vitamin, some of the early
signs may be apparent, such as roughening and
symmetrical discoloration of the skin, especially of
the face. It is wise at this stage, even if pellagra is not
the disease, to take a course of nicotinic acid and

revise your diet.

Children on an inadequate diet, who feel tired and sleepy in school and seem to lack intelligence, are halfway to pellagra. They can be cured by an all round diet of plenty of fresh vegetables, wholemeal bread, brewer's yeast, yeast extract, liver (or liver extracts) and fish, such as salmon, herring and cod. The same, of course, applies to adults. It is better to eat well than resort to medicaments.

CHAPTER SIX

VITAMIN B2 OR RIBOFLAVIN

Not till 1926 did scientists know for certain that the vitamin they called B was really many vitamins all rolled into one, and that the various parts, when broken down and isolated, would cure diseases unrelated to each other.

Originally the B-complex was called B2 (in America G, in honour of Goldberger), because at one time it was thought that B2, or riboflavin was the cure for pellagra. But, as explained, it is nicotinic acid that does the trick.

For years men have suffered from a disease called cheilosis or ariboflavinosis (without riboflavin), without knowing how it was caused or how it could be cured. Shortly before the Second World War scientists discovered that cheilosis could be induced by depriving the system of riboflavin (B2).

In cheilosis, facial skin reddens and cracks at the edges of the mouth; lips and tongue grow abnormally red; skin at the folds between nostrils and cheeks becomes greasy and sheds; and the corners of the eyes and underneaths of the eyelids grow sore. In extreme cases cataracts sprout over the lenses of the eyes. In India millions who live on food deficient in B2 develop cataract, which now can be arrested by taking B2.

Foods rich in riboflavin are yeast (the best source), fresh raw milk, leafy green vegetables such as beet, turnip and carrot tops, broccoli, spinach, lettuce and cabbage and the germ and bran of wheat.

Often women who suffer from cracked, rough skin use expensive face creams to 'feed' it, whereas what they really need is much more vitamin B2 in their food. If they will only eat 100 per cent wholemeal bread and never white, drink plenty of milk (or skim milk), have an egg or two every day and plenty of salads and cooked greens they will observe a startling improvement. Instead, through ignorance they clog their pores with costly grease and continue to eat foods denuded of both minerals and vitamins.

Whole wheat and whole rye are excellent foods and furnish the entire B-complex family. If a handful of wheat is soaked in warm water, spread on a board one layer thick and then covered with a napkin wrung out in warm water and left for two days and nights in a warm place, it will sprout and develop vitamin C. Pour milk over this sprouting grain and eat it, and if you add a herring to this simple dish you will get all the vitamins you need.

You don't have to dine at the Ritz to get all the nourishment your body needs, or visit the chemist for your vitamins; you can get them all for a few pence at home.

Another well-balanced meal is wholemeal bread (B-complex and E); butter (A, B1 and D); a baked potato (C); fresh salad (mainly A and C); milk (A, B and D); and herrings (A, B and D); and these foods will also supply proteins, carbohydrates and fat and an abundance of the minerals, calcium and phosphorous.

The food you can get at home is nearly always better and richer than that you buy in cafés and restaurants, which is often refined and denuded of life-giving properties. If you eat out and demand brown bread you will get, at best, bread of 85 per cent extraction or a wheat-germ loaf with the bran extracted; sugar that is white (rarely Demerara, Barbados or Muscavados); polished rice and edibles that have been kept in cold store for days, weeks and even months. A poulterer friend confided to me that he keeps turkeys sometimes for two years, returning them to store if he fails to get rid of them at Christmas. The protein in such birds may not have diminished, but the vitamins undoubtedly have.

According to Professor Ida Mann of Oxford University and her colleague Dr Antoinette Pirie, who together have done considerable research on the eyes, B_2 is vital for healthy eyes and good sight. There are, for instance, no blood vessels in the cornea. The tiny blood vessels from the conjunctiva normally stop at the junction of the cornea and sclera, or white of the eye. But if there is a deficiency of riboflavin in the system the blood vessels from the conjunctiva grow into the cornea and may even continue to the area of the pupil. Opaque spots appear in the cornea and the eye grows inflamed and sore.

Wholemeal bread, beer and tea (our national beverage) all contain riboflavin, so, if wholemeal bread and one of these beverages is imbibed, this condition should vanish.

CHAPTER SEVEN

VITAMIN B12

Next, there is B12, a relatively recent addition to the family; the vitamin that holds out hope to all anaemics. Anaemia occurs when the blood is deficient in red blood corpuscles or haemoglobin, or both.

At first, in Europe, iron was the specific for anaemia, though advanced cases did not respond. But in China since time immemorial, liver was always given to those who suffered from anaemia.

Kenneth Walker tells us in *The Story of Blood* of an English lady in China who suffered from severe anaemia. As European doctors could do nothing for her she took the advice of her maid and consulted a Chinese healer, who gave her some pills, which quickly restored her to health. When she asked what the pills were made of the doctor said that he employed a small boy to shoot crows and it was from their livers that the pills were concocted!

Whereas ordinary anaemia could be cured by iron either in solid or liquid form, 'pernicious anaemia' could not, and for a doctor to say that a patient had this disease was tantamount to a sentence of death.

Blood contains both red and white corpuscles, the red vastly predominating. These are manufactured in the most carefully protected areas of the body, namely, the interiors of the bones, particularly the long bones and ribs.

About 55 years ago Dr George Minot, an American, decided to find out why, in the cases of anaemic persons, red blood corpuscles were no longer manufactured in the marrow, and how this destructive process could be arrested.

He discovered in 1921 that without exception, victims of pernicious anaemia also suffered from a wasting of the stomach and a wasting of blood. Then, *he* started wasting, but his condition was diagnosed as diabetes and shots of insulin enabled him to continue his researches.

His interest in diet was stimulated and when Dr Whipple, one of the pioneers in the study of blood, suggested that pernicious anaemia might be caused by the lack of some substance that forms the red cells, Minot's nose bent to the trail.

In 1924 he induced a colleague, Dr Bill Murphy, to treat anaemic patients by making them eat half-a-pound of raw liver every day as well as a quarter pound of lean meat. In two years 45 patients on this nauseating diet all recovered. This was an unprecedented achievement, and so great was their contribution to human welfare that Minot, Murphy and Whipple were awarded a Nobel Prize for their endeavours.

The Intrinsic Factor
They decided that pernicious anaemia was caused by the immobilization or lack of some enzyme created in the stomach which prevents the digestive organs from converting iron into red blood corpuscles, and that extracts from the stomachs of healthy animals (or liver extracts) enabled this element, which they termed the 'intrinsic factor', to function.

It is now known from research carried out by the Agricultural Department of the University of Michigan that the cow manufactures this intrinsic factor in her rumen, but she will fail to produce it in her milk if traces of cobalt are absent from the soil in which her feed is grown, and ultimately become anaemic, cease eating and die.

In 1948 Mrs Mary S. Shorb of the Maryland Agricultural Experimental Station and her colleague Dr Folkers, and a team of scientists led by Dr Lester Smith in Greenford, England, claimed simultaneously to have found this missing factor, a vitamin containing cobalt, which they named B12. It is the only vitamin to contain a mineral element, and cobalt is one of those 'trace elements' about which we are learning more each year. They appear in minute quantities in the soil, but, if missing, those who eat food grown in such soil suffer from diseases which have hitherto baffled doctors.

'Pernicious anaemics' are now treated with injections of from 10 to 100 micrograms of B12. A microgram is one thousandth part of a milligram, or a millionth part of a gram. Thus, a microgram is equal to one twenty-eighth of a millionth part of an ounce avoirdupois!

Not only does B12 restore the constituents of the blood to normal, it improves the general well-being of the patient; and once the disease is under control doses of from 1-3 micrograms daily, or 10 once a fortnight, are sufficient.

Vegetarians who, on principle, object to liver or liver injections containing B12 need not be dismayed; they, too, can be cured, for it was later discovered that a mould, *Streptomyces griseus*, is rich in B12, and immeasurably greater quantities of the vitamin can be manufactured from this source at a much smaller cost, than from liver. In fact, B12 is no longer extracted from liver, for it takes 20 tons of liver to produce one gram of B12!

Incidentally, the complete structure of B12 was not known till 1948, when the constituents were discovered simultaneously by an American group at the Merck Laboratories in New Jersey, Mrs D.C. Hodgkin at Oxford, Sir Alexander Dodd at Cambridge, scientists at the Glaxo Laboratories, Greenford, and workers at the University of California.

CHAPTER EIGHT

VITAMIN E

Scientists are discovering new uses for vitamin E every year. We know that if vitamin E is lacking, females fail to carry their young and males can be rendered sterile. It prevents abortions and miscarriages, and during the menopause helps to banish hot flushes, depression, sweating, fear and nervousness.

Dr Evan Shute and Dr Vogelsang, pioneers in vitamin E therapy, have immeasurably improved the condition of patients suffering from weak heart and have relieved swollen feet, ankles and legs, breathlessness and stabbing pains with large doses of wheat germ oil (*alpha-tocopherol*). This gives increased oxygen consumption and Dr A.M. Pappenheimer says that it alters the metabolism of the muscular tissues, bringing relief.

Dr Shute says that vitamin E improves the circulation and phlebitis and varicose veins respond to treatment 'by producing collateral circulation about the obstructed deep veins and calling into play the great unused network of veins lying in wait for emergencies'.

No one who invariably eats 100 per cent wholemeal bread and supplements his diet with wheat germ need suffer a scarcity of vitamin E, but unfortunately millions live on bread, steamed puddings, pastries and biscuits made from white flour – from which the germ of the wheat has been extracted – and are sadly lacking in this essential element.

Incidentally, in Russia, vitamins A, E and K are being made from cheap materials into a substance called *citral* which is fed daily to cattle and poultry and when results have been established will, in all probability, be available to humans.